NCLEX
Nuggets

NCLEX
Nuggets

A Compilation
of
Study Notes
for the NCLEX Exam

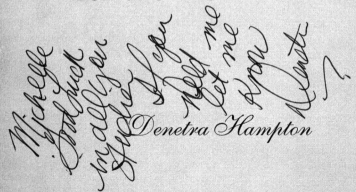

Denetra Hampton

Copyright © 2009 by Denetra Hampton.

Library of Congress Control Number:		2009901080
ISBN:	Hardcover	978-1-4415-0758-7
	Softcover	978-1-4415-0757-0

This book was printed in the United States of America.

To order additional copies of this book, contact:
Xlibris Corporation
1-888-795-4274
www.Xlibris.com
Orders@Xlibris.com
57258

DEDICATION

TO GOD WHO IS ABLE TO KEEP YOU FROM FALLING . . . .

IN MEMORY OF MY MOTHER WHO INSTILLED IN ME THE
CONFIDENCE

TO PURSUE MY DREAMS . . . .

TO ALL THE GRADUATE NURSES WHO ARE PREPARING TO
PASS THE NCLEX EXAM . . .

CONTENTS

BOOK SUMMARY STATEMENT

THE NCLEX EXAM FOR REGISTERED NURSES IS THE FINAL
DETERMINENT OF
THE GRADUATE NURSES EDUCATION AND ABILITY TO
PRACTICE PROFESSIONALLY. THIS HANDBOOK IS A TOOL
DEVELOPED TO ASSIST THE GRADUATE NURSE IN STUDYING
FOR THIS VERY IMPORTANT EXAM.
THE CONTENT WAS DEVELOPED TO ENHANCE THE STUDY-
HABITS OF THE GRADUATE NURSE WHILE PROVIDING
DIRECTION AND DISCIPLINE FOR THOSE WHO ARE HAVING
DIFFICULTY PASSING THE NCLEX EXAM.
AS NURSES WE ARE GUIDED BY THE PRINCIPLE, "EACH ONE
TEACH ONE".
THIS IS THE SAME PRINCIPLE THAT DIRECTED THIS PROJECT.
BY REACHING BACK WE HELP OUR SOCIETY AND FELLOW
COLLEGUES PROVIDE AND MAINTAIN QUALITY CARE.
GOOD LUCK!

THE AUTHOR

Denetra Hampton was born in Paris, Texas. She graduated from Hampton University with her Bachelor of Science in Nursing, received her Masters of Health Administration and is currently enrolled in a Doctorate degree program.

She has worked in the nursing specialties of Orthopedics, Medical-Surgical, Post Anesthesia, and is currently working in an Intensive Care Unit. She has served the nursing community as a nursing school clinical instructor and continues to serve the profession through education.

Denetra has been married to her husband Shawn for 13 years, they have one four-legged child, Fancy.

PART I

Test-Taking Strategies and Preparation

Picture yourself taking care of the patient!

Identify key words such as: "most correct, most likely, do first, highest priority"

- Early and Late symptoms

- Most or Least likely to occur

- Initial means first (think assessment)

- Essential means safety (YOU HAVE TO DO THIS!)

- Remember : Keep them BREATHING and Keep them SAFE!

If two answers say the same thing in different words they are both incorrect; Example: poor appetite and anorexia mean the same

Words from the question are repeated in the answer

Longer answers are usually correct

Odd man wins in nursing

What is the question asking?

Delegation and Supervision Strategy

- Patients Bill of Rights

- Nurse Practice Act

- Make sure the task is one you can delegate

  Can the person perform the task

  Is it LEGAL to delegate it to the person

Delegate stable patients and unchanging procedures

  ex: bathing, feeding

Do not delegate assessment activites

When deciding priorities always use MASLOW's, NURSING Process and SAFETY.

Priority Strategy

- Who should you visit/see FIRST

  Stability

  Is the situation "acute"

  Is there an assessment to be done

  Immediate attention

Remember therapeutic communication

If the question is asking you to assess, ASSESS, if the answer has one thing in it that is not assessment it is wrong

If "Best answer" is in the question; discrimination is involved

If the question asks you to use an "Intravenous" medication, the answer will be the medication that indicates I.V.

Know that the information given is the only information, do not guess or add your own input

Go with your first instinct

Know the step of the *Nursing process* that is being tested

Assessment words: observe, assess, recognize, collect

Analysis words: diagnose, define, order, and sort

Planning words: rearrange, include, outcome

Implementation words: inform, document, explain, administer

Evaluation words: monitor, repeat, and demonstrate

Avoid choices with the words, "always, never, all, or none"

Always go with ABC's

Look at relationship between answers

Look for the shortest or longest answer

Concentrate on words in the questions such as: acute, post-op, most immediate

Re-read two answers that seem the same; there is some difference between them

Review content

Practice Multiple-choice questions

Practice stress reducers

Respect the NCLEX Exam

Set-up a study schedule

Develop flash cards

Overlearn the material

Keep a positive, confident attitude before taking the test and following the test

Review the NCLEX test plan

PART II

Respiratory Notes

Breathing Patterns

Tachypnea-increased rate (anxiety)

Bradypnea—decreased rate (coma)

Kussmal—deep, rapid respirations (DKA)

Cheyne-Stokes—cycles of rapid breaths (ICP)

Orthopnea—inability to lie flat (CHF)

Paroxysmal Nocturnal Dypsnea—SOB after lying flat

Stridor—crowing sound

Breath Sounds

Bronchial—high-pitched located over trachea)

Bronchovesicular—medium pitched (located in airways)

Vesicular—low-pitched (located in lung fields)

Bronchial or bronchovesicular sounds heard over lungs may be Pneumonia

Adventitious Sounds

Crackles—bubbling sounds (COPD)

Wheezes—musical sounds (asthma)

Rubs—grating sound (pleura inflammation)

Sputum

Rust—pneumonia

Pink and frothy—pulmonary edema

Greenish—acute bronchitis

Arterial Blood Gases

Norms

Ph   7.35-7.45

Pc02 35 to 45

Hc03 24-30

P02   80-100

	Ph	pc02	Hc03
Respiratory acidosis	↓	↑	N (COPD)
Respiratory alkalosis (HYPERVENTILATION)	↑	↓	N
Metabolic acidosis (DKA)	↓	N	↓
Metabolic alkalosis (VOMITING)	↑	N	↑

Oxygen Delivery Systems

Nasal Cannula—delivers low Oxygen levels of 24-40% (6 LPM)

Face Mask-delivers oxygen levels of 30-60% (4-6 LMP)

NON-rebreather—high concentrations of (50-100%)

Suctioning

Conscious patient—semi-fowlers

Unconscious patient—on side

Apply suction no longer than 10 seconds and only suction during withdrawal of catheter

Oral—catheter no deeper than the distance from ear lobe to the tip of the nose

Tracheal—catheter no deeper than 6 to 12 inches (pre-oxygenate with 100% oxygen)

Trach Care

Tie all ties with a knot and never cut old ties until new ties are in place

Trach cuffs have no more than 3 ml of air in them

Always have emergency equipment at the bedside i.e.(trach set)

Chest Tubes

Removes air or fluid

Used after pneumothorax or chest surgery to re-expand lung

Absence of bubbling in the suction control chamber means suction not being maintained

Absence of bubbling in the water seal chamber indicated lung expansion

If the patient becomes SOB after clamping the chest tube, there is still air in the spaces

Removal of a chest tube is done at the end of a inspiration (instruct patient to exhale and bear down)

Three chamber system

Suction—should bubble vigorously

Water seal—should not bubble; fluctuates with respirations

Drainage—collects blood; should not be greater than 100ml/hr

Water seal is bubbling: check for air leak

Bronchoscopy

Pre-procedure

Informed consent

NPO for 8 hours prior

Administer atropine as directed to dry secretions

Tonsillectomy

Difficulty swallowing post-op

Post-op hemorrhage can occur

Monitor for continuous swallowing

Pneumonia

Antibiotics

CDB

Fluids

Semi-Fowlers position

Tuberculosis

Spread by Airborne droplets

BCG vaccine

Positive PPD (read in 48-72 hours)

5 tuberculin units

PPD is positive if 10mm or more, raised and red

Immunosuppressed patients will be positive at 5mm; treat with INH, rifampin, ethambutal, streptomycin; medications taken for 9 months

Pulmonary Embolism

Post-op inactivity

Bed rest

DVT

Sit patient in high-fowlers

Oxygen in high rate via mask

ABG

Administer anticoagulants

Restlessness is a sign of acute respiratory distress

COPD

Asthma, Bronchitis, Emphysema

Cough, wheezing, and dypsnea

Six small meals a day

Avoid Chest PT 1 hour before and 1 hour after meals

Pursed lip breathing

Patient should stay away from crowds

Right sided heart failure

Albuterol is a bronchodilator used with COPD

ARDS

    Dyspnea, tachypnea, grunting, flaring nostrils, cyanosis

    Mechanical ventilation

    Albumin used to decrease pulmonary edema

    Steroids for inflammation

    Diuretics to decrease fluid overload

Pneumothorax

    closed=sharp pain, dyspnea, shock

    open= sucking noise, tracheal deviation to affected side

    tension= tracheal deviation to unaffected side

    Absent or diminished breath sounds over collapsed lung

Thoracotomy

    Pneumonectomy= whole lung/ position on operative side or back

    Lobectomy= part of lung/ position on back or either side

    ICS

    Frozen shoulder syndrome may be a complication/ ROM exercises

NCLEX Nuggets

When suctioning a patient with a tracheostomy tube always assemble the equipment FIRST

After a bronchoscopy pink-tinged sputum is normal, but bright red blood indicates hemorrhage

Symptoms of a closed pneumothorax are SOB, and chest pain

Positions that help with breathing are sitting up, leaning over a able and standing Up against a wall

TB is spread via airborne route

Pursed lip breathing gives the maximum expiration for patients with COPD

Earliest sign of ARDS is tachypnea

Common signs of Pulmonary Embolism are tachypnea, dyspnea, and chest pain

When using a metered dose inhaler, shake the can, hold it upright, inhale, and deliver one spray per breath

Emphysema, leads to "barrel chest"

Pulmonary Sarcoidosis includes dry cough, dyspnea, and hemoptysis. It is treated with corticosteroids

Low PaO2 levels trigger breathing in a patient with emphysema

Increased PaO2 levels trigger breathing in a normal respiratory drive

Asthma is caused by sensitivity to allergens such as pollen, dust and dander

Basis gas exchange in the lungs is the alveoli

Surfactant reduces surface tension to keep alveoli from collapsing

During flail chest a portion of the chest wall moves in during inspiration which creates a paradoxical chest movement

Subcutaneous emphysema is found in the patient with tension pneumothorax

After a pneumonectomy place the patient on his back or affected side

Disappearance of wheeze in acute conditions may be an airway obstruction

Best position for a patient with respiratory problems is HIGH Fowlers

Sputum culture is the definitive test for TB

Inspiratory and expiratory wheezes are findings in asthma

Bronchodilators are the first line of treatment for asthma

COPD patients are considered "blue bloaters" and Emphysema patients are considered "pink puffers"

Diuretics are used for COPD patients

In ARDS the alveoli are filled with fluid

PEEP (positive-end-expiratory pressure) reduces cardiac output by increasing intrathoracic pressure

SOB and absent breath sounds on the right side are indicative of a spontaneoud pneumothorax

An indication of lung re-expnasion is the loss of fluctuation in the water seal chamber when suction is not applied

Ambulate early to reduce pulmonary embolism

Heparin is started when a pulmonary embolism has been diagnosed

CARDIOVASCULAR NOTES

Blood Flow

Blood follows this sequence through the heart: superior and inferior vena cava → right atrium → tricuspid valve → right ventricle → pulmonary semilunar valve → pulmonary trunk and arteries to the lungs → pulmonary veins leaving the lungs → left atrium → bicuspid valve → left ventricle → aortic semilunar valve → aorta → to the body.

Atherosclerosis is due to a build-up of fatty material (*plaque*), mainly cholesterol, under the inner lining of arteries. The plaque can cause a *thrombus* (blood clot) to form. The thrombus can dislodge as an *embolus* and lead to *thromboembolism*

Rate and Rhythm

NORMAL SINUS RHUTM—60-100 BPM

SINUS BRADYCARDIA—less than 60 BPM

SINUS TACHYCARDIA—greater than 100BPM

Discolorations

Pallor

Cyanosis

Edema

Treatments

ECG-P wave, QRS complex, T wave,

Stress Test—measures symptoms and cardiac changes occurring with cardiac diseases; Patient walks on treadmill or rides bike

Holter Monitor

Used to measure heart rates and rhythms over prolonged periods of time, usually 24 hours

Cardiac catherization

Dye may be salty or metallic taste when injected

Patients may have nausea with dye injection

No aspirin or aspirin like products for 7 days prior to procedure

Angina

P= palliative	Pain caused by activity/relieved
Q= quality	Heavy, crushing, dull
R= region	Over sternum, epigastric area, jaw, back, shoulders
S= severity	Mild to severe
T = timing	Usually related to activity or stress

ECG have T wave changes

Nitroglycerin used to increase oxygen perfusion

Headache is the most common side effect of Nitroglycerine

Myocardial Infarction

Typical MI Pain

P = No relation to activity and no relief from meds

Q = Heavy, crushing, dull

R = Over sternum, epigastric area, jaw, back, shoulders

S = Mild to severe, feeling of doom, N/V; diaphoresis, pallor

T = lasts longer than 15 minutes

Dysrhymias are the most common complication associated with an MI

CPK, LDH, and SGOT/AST are cardiac enzymes that help diagnose an MI

Management of MI includes oxygen and morphine

Congestive Heart Failure

Right-sided failure reveals systemic symptoms

    peripheral edema of extremities

    jugular vein distention

    hepatomegaly

    splenomegaly

    ascites

Left sided failure reveals respiratory symptoms

    SOB

    orthopnea

    crackles in both lungs

    oliguria

Management Aldactone, lasix Digoxin

Digoxin Therapy

    Anti-arrhythmic agent; increases C/O and slows heart rate withhold dose if pulse is < 60

    bradycardia

    halo

N/V

anorexia

Assess for:

Heart rate, Dig level, K+

NCLEX Nuggets

Cheyne-Stokes respirations—noted for apneic periods; left ventricular failure

Ateclectasis—collapse of alveoli or lobule; associated with pleural effusion or pneumothorax

Hemoptsis—indicative of pulmonary edema; pink or blood-tinged frothy sputum

Rales—noted at bases of lungs; associated w/ CHF

Tachypnea—rapid, shallow breathing associated w/ CHF

Wheezes—compression of small airways; associated w/ pulmonary edema

Purpose of water in the water seal chamber of a chest tube is to prevent the entrance of air into the pleural cavity

Pulmonary Edema

Abnormal collection of fluid in lungs

pink sputum

restlessness

cyanosis

SOB

Rales

cold skin

Management

    Monitor blood pressure

    Oxygen

    Sit patient up

    Total care

    Diuretics

Cardiogenic Shock: Heart loses its contractility; inadequate tissue perfusion; end stage of heart failure

low blood pressure

Rapid pulse

Confusion

Dysrhythmias

Hypoxia

Oliguria

Decreases CO

An acute MI causes cardiogenic shock

Other disease processes you should know are :

    Aortic insufficiency—incomplete closure of valves

    Cardiomyopathy—disease of the muscle

    Infective endocarditis—infection of the valves

    Mitral stenosis—incomplete emptying of left atrium

Pericarditis—inflammation of membranous sac; pain most common symptom with friction rub

Rheumatic endocarditis—results from nodules that lead to scarring; strep infection

Cardiac Tamponade

Blood or fluid in pericardial sac

distant heart sounds

jugular venous distention

paradoxical pulse

dyspnea

Cyanotic Heart Disease

created by a right-to-left shunt

Tetra logy of Fallot

Cyanosis and fatigue

Child finds relief in squat position

Acyanotic Heart disease

Blood shunts left-to-right through opening

Patent Ductus Arteriosis

Poor feeding

poor growth

respiratory infections

Rhematic Fever

history of strep infection

Pregnancy-Induced Hypertension (PIIH)

After 20th week

edema around eyes and face, proteinuria

hypertension; increase of 30 mm systolic/ 15mm diastolic

Deep vein thrombosis

Calf pain, redness, warmth to touch over area positive homan's

sign; potential for PE

Administration of Heparin(monitor PTT)remember two t's make an "H"

NCLEX Nuggets

A modified lifestyle is the first step in the treatment of hypertension

The key to ventricular fibrillation treatment is early defibrillation and CPR

Aspirin should not be taken at least 7 days prior to surgery to reduce the risk of postoperative bleeding

Cardiogenic shock is a condition of diminished cardiac output

Dopamine increases cardiac output

the left anterior descending artery is the source of blood for the anterior wall of the heart

Cholesterol levels above 200mg/dl are considered excessive

Increasing oxygen is always the first intervention when a patient exhibits signs of cardiac compromise

The left fifth intercostals space at the midclavicular line is the landmark for the apical pulse

CK-MB enzymes are present after an MI

Supplemental potassium is given with furosemide because of its potassium-sparing effects

When the left ventricle does not function properly left sided heart failure results; fluid accumulates in the interstitial spaces and alveolar spaces in the lungs and this causes crackles

An echocardiogram is used to view myocardial wall function

The green halo sign is the most common sign if digoxin toxicity

A pulsating abdominal mass indicates a abdominal aortic aneurysm

Marfan's syndrome results from degeneration of the elastic fibers

Unstable angina progressively increases in frequency,intensity and duration

Nitroglycerine is the drug of choice for angina pectoris

Earliest sign of cardiogenic shock is altered LOC

Kidneys respond to hypertension by excreting sodium and excess water

The bell of the stethoscope is placed over the brachial artery to obtain a blood pressure

Varicose veins normally occur in the saphenous veins

Chest tubes are used to return negative pressure to the intrapleural space and expand the lungs

HEMATOLOGY NOTES

Red blood cells—formed in bone marrow

White blood cells—formed in bone marrow and lymphatic tissue

Plasma—liquid part of blood

Spleen-filters blood; administer Vitamin k before a splenectomy

Liver—largest organ in the body—produces bile, metabolizes carbs, fats, and proteins

Type A people can receive A or O blood

Type B people can receive B or O blood

Type O people receive O blood only

Neutrophils = bacterial infection

Eosinophils = allergies

Basophils = inflammation

Lymphocytes = viral infection

Monocytes = infections

Blood Transfusions

physicians order

typed & cross

normal saline

obtain V/S every 5 minutes for first 15 minutes

If reaction stop blood transfusion

Types = hemolytic, allergic, bacterial

Pernicious Anemia

vitamin b12 deficiency

tingling and numbness, gait abnormalities red beefy tongue

diagnosed by schilling test

Sickle Cell anemia

Predominantly black populations

inherited genetic disorder

crisis triggered by infection, dehydration, high altitudes

management of crisis: increase fluids; pain meds

Thalassemia: Colley's anemia

genetic disorder in children

enlarged spleen, cachexia, jaundice

Hemolytis disease in Pregnancy

RH negative and ABO incompatibility (mother RH neg; father positive; baby positive

Mother must get Rhogam within 72 hours

Hemophilia

inherited X-link recessive bleeding disorder; (missing clotting factor VIII)

    carried on X chromosome; manifested in male

    manage with replacement of factor VIII (cryoprecipitate)

Lead Poisoning

    reaction to ingestion of lead substances

    chelating agents given orally, IV or IM

Leukemia

    uncontrolled proliferation of WBC precursors

    bruising, bleeding, bone pain, lethargy

    chemotherapy; radiation therapy

Neutropenic Precautions

A private room is recommended

Neutropenic precautionary sign

Educate family members

Use of PPE

If have mild upper respiratory infections must wear mask

If have GI or skin infections do not care for this type of patient

No live plants or flowers

NCLEX Nuggets

Always monitor the Potassium level when giving Digoxin and Lasix

Ventricular Tachycardia is seen with no P waves, wide QRS complexes and 100-300 Heart rate; treatment is lidocaine and or cardioversion

Therapeutic range for PT is 1.5 2 times the control for high risk thrombus patients

Always apply 5 minutes of pressure to the site after an ABG

Homan's Sign indicates thrombophlebitis

Lavage removes blood from the stomach

The most severe complication from anticoagulation is hemorrhage

NEUROLOGIC NOTES

Autonomic Nervous System

Sympathetic	Parasympathetic
Flight or flight	Maintains normal body function
Increases heart rate/ BP	Normalizes heart rate/BP
Increases RR	Normalizes RR
Decreases peristalsis	Increases peristalsis
Secretes epinephrine/ norepinephrine	Secretes acetylcholine
Dialate bronchioles	Constricts bronchioles

Cranial Nerves

I	Olfactory	Smell	On
II	Optic	Vision	old
III	Oculomotor	Extraocular movements	Olympus
IV	Trochlear	Extraocular movements	Towering
V	Trigeminal	Pain, touch, chewing	Tops
VI	Abducens	Extraocular movements	A
VII	Facial	Taste, close eyes, smile, puff cheeks	finn
VIII	acoustic	Hearing	And
IX	Glosso-pharyngeal	Taste, gag, swallow	German
X	Vagus	Gag and swallow	Viewed
XI	accessory	Shoulder and neck strength	A
XII	hypoglossal	Stick out tongue	hop

Brain

Frontal lobe—personality

Parietal Lobe—sensation

Temporal lobe—hearing

Occipital Lobe—vision

cerebellum—coordination of muscle groups

ontanel—interpretation of sensation

Hypothalmus—temperature control

Gait abnormalities

scissors gate—paraplegia

hemiplegia gait—arm rigid/leg on same side not easily lifted

Ataxic gait—loss of position sense/ wide stand

Propulsive/retropulsive—patient moves as if going to fall forward; Parkinson disease

LOC—best indicator of neurological status

Glasco Coma Scale

eye opening

best motor response

best verbal response

Cushing's Triad

increased systolic pressure

Widening pulse pressure

bradycardia

decreased respiratory rate

Decorticate—arms turned in and up; toward the cortex

Decerebrate—rigid extension; arms fully extended; forearms pronated

Expressive aphasia—inability to speak

receptive aphasia—inability to understand

Cerebellar function—includes evaluation of balance and coordination

Romberg's test—patient stands erect with feet together, first with eyes open and then closed;

NCLEX Nuggets

— If unable to maintain balance this is *ROMBERG'S SIGN* and indicates damage

— Deep tendon reflex—knee tap

— Babinski reflex—sole of foot is stroked from heel to ball of foot, toes should curl downward; if not, POSITIVE BABINSKI SIGN

— Wernicke's syndrome is a degenerative neurological disorder associated with alcohol ingestion and thiamine deficiency

— Guillain-Barre syndrome is usually preceded by a viral infection

Seizure Disorders

Seizure	Assessment
Tonic-clonic	Aura,loc,rigidity,repetitive limb movement postictal lethargy
Petit-mal	Brief LOC,twitching or rolling of eyes
Myoclonic	Brief spasm of a single muscle group
Atonic	Sudden loss of muscle tone brief loss of LOC
Simple	Motor, sensory, autonomic deficits w/o LOC
Complex	Cognitive, psychosensory,preceded by aura

Maintain safety at all times

Do not stick anything in the patient's mouth

Dilantin (10-20mcg/ml)

Phenobarbital

Tegretol

Right sided CVA

brain damage with symptoms on the left side

left sided neglect

left sided Hemianopsia (

ontanel patient from unaffected side)

left hemiplegia

Left sided CVA

brain damage with symptoms on right side

expressive aphasia

receptive aphasia

communication is major problem

unable to ambulate (stand on unaffected side to assist)

A cane is used on the unaffected side and is advanced just before or at the same time as the affected leg is moved forward

Tensilon test

Used to diagnose Myasthenia Gravis

Autonomic dysreflexia

occurs at T-6 level

sudden headache; increase of systolic blood pressure

Hypertension

Distended bladder; fecal impaction

Multiple Sclerosis

Weakness

nystagmus

diplopia

paresthesia

blurred vision

impaired sensation

paralysis

optic neuritis

Management of MS

plasmapheresis

muscle relaxant

glucocorticoids

immunosuppressants

skeletal muscle relaxants

Myasthenia gravis

neuromuscular disorder

weakness of voluntary muscles

muscle weakness increases with activity and decreases with rest

Management of Myasthenia gravis

neostigimine

glucocorticoids

immunosuppressants

antineoplastics

Guillian Barre' syndrome

peripheral polyneuritis

characterized by ascending paralysis

respiratory paralysis

Management of Guillian Barre' syndrome

plasmapheresis

nutritional support

Glucocorticoids

Meningitis

inflammation of the brain and spinal cord meninges caused by bacterial infection fever, chills, tachycardia, petechial rash, nuchal rigidity, Positive Brudzinski's sign

Management of meningitis

I.V. therapy

oxygen

antibiotics

diuretics

anticonvulsants

Bell's palsy

blocked cranial nerve VII

unilateral facial weakness

pain around jaw or ear

Management of Bell's palsy

Heat and corticosteroids

NCLEX Nuggets

To prevent an increase in ICP elevate the HOB 30 to 40 degrees

Alzheimer's is characterized by progressive degeneration of the cerebral cortex

Epilepsy is characterized by involuntary muscle contractions

Guilliane Barre' is characterized by ascending paralysis

Stroke is characterized by sensory and motor deficits caused by a disruption of cerebral circulation

Eating problems associated with Parkinson include aspiration, choking, constipation, and dysphagia

Heachache following a lumbar puncture is usually caused by CSF leak

Light flashes and floaters are characteristics of a detached retina

Disabling glare is a symptom of cataracts

Eye pain, halo vision and redness are characteristic of angle-closure-glaucoma

Aspirin, streptomycin and neomycin are associated with ototoxicity

Types of cells

T-cells lymphocytes

B-cells

T-killer cells, T-helper cells, T-suppressor cells

Immunoglobulin

IgM. IgA, IgG, IgD, Ig E

HIV

Low WBC

T4 cell count less than 300mmmm

Positive Elisa test

Kaposi's Sarcoma,PCP pneumonia,AZT,PPD test is positive with 5mm or more indurated

Rheumatoid Arthritis

Inflammation of synovial membranes and joints that leads to deformities and loss of joint function

— Persistent joint pain lasting > 3 months

— Morning stiffness

— Restricted ROM on affected joints

— Positive RF factor, Elevated ESR

NCLEX Nuggets

Bone marrow serves as a positive diagnostic predictor for immunologic disorders.

Cell-mediated immunity is responsible for the mediation of transplant rejection.

Coombs blood test can define the presence of hemolytic anemia

Mental status changes is the most frequent sign of infection in an older adult

Epinephrine is the drug of choice for anaphylaxis

Plaquenil is an antimalarial agent used in the treatment of rheumatoid arthritis

Raynaud's phenomenon is one of the most common findings in systemic sclerosis

GASTROINTESTINAL NOTES

Types of Pain

Appendix—lower quandrant w/ rebound tenderness (McBurney;s Point) Right lower quandrant

Cholecystitis—upper right quandrant and right shoulder

Murphy's sign—palpation during inspiration creates pain and inability to take a deep breath

Pancreatitis—mid-epigastric and radiating to back or left shoulder

Diverticulitis—lower left quandrant pain

Aspirin is irritating to the gastric mucosa and is known to cause ulcers

Preparation for a GI series:

NPO 8 hours

Barium swallow

Differences between Gastric and Duodenal ulcers

	Gastric ulcer	Duodenal ulcer
Age	Over 65	Under 65
Sex prevalence	Female	Male
Family history	Yes	no
Risk factors	Stress, smoking, ETOH	
Location	Stomach antrum	Proximal 1-2 cm of the duodenum
Signs	Upper abdominal pain 1-2 hours after eating; aggravated by food	Upper abdominal pain 2-4 hours after eating; relieved by food
Course	Chronic and weight loss	Cyclical occurrences with exacerbations; weight gain

Post-operative complication of Gastric resection surgery

Dumping syndrome—palpitations, dizziness, weakness, abdominal cramping, instruct patient to eat 6 small, dry feedings per day that are high in carbs rest for 30 min following meals

Parotitis—is usually caused by prolonged NPO status

BRAT DIET—used in children for vomiting and diarrhea

bananas, rice, applesauce, toast

Hirschsprung's disease—decreased mobility in large bowel; distended abdomen

TPN

Catheter site changed every 4 weeks

IV tubing and filters changed every 24 hours

Dressing changed 2-3 times a week and PRN

The patient with pancreatitis should eat small frequent meals

Peptic Ulcer

left epigastric pain for 1-2 hours

hematemesis

relief of pain after antacids

Management of Peptic ulcer

antibiotics

surgery

Ulcerative Colitis

inflammation of the large bowel

viral and bacterial infections

weight loss, abdominal cramping, bloody stools,

hyperactive bowel sounds

Management of Ulcerative Colitis

I.V. therapy

antibiotics

Antiemetics

anti-inflammatory agents

Chron's disease

inflammatory disease of the small intestine

effects the terminal ileum

usually the ascending colon

pain in right lower quandrant, abdominal cramps and spasms

after meals, chronic bloody diarrhea

diagnosed with classic "string sign" at terminal ileum

"cobblestone" appearance of intestinal mucosa

Management of Chron's disease

antibiotics, antidiarrheals, anti-inflammatory agents

Diverticulitis

outpouching of intestinal mucosa

low intake of fiber

stress

chronic constipation

Left lower quadrant pain, bloody stools, nausea

Management of Diverticulitis

high fiber diet, antibiotics, stool softeners

Peritonitis

inflammation of the peritoneal cavity

bacterial infection

abdominal pain, rebound tenderness, fever, abdominal rigidity,

decreased or absent bowel sounds

Management of Peritonitis

I.V. therapy, NG tube, antibiotics, withhold food and fluids

Cholecystitis

acute or chronic inflammation of the gallbladder

obesity, infection of the gallbladder, indigestion or chest pain, episodic colicky pain in the epigastric area that radiates to back and shoulder, jaundice

Management of Cholesystitis

low fat diet, vitamins, withhold food and fluids

Pancreatitis

inflammation of the pancreas

alcoholism, hyperparathyroidism, hyperlipidemia

nausea and vomiting, tachycardia, pain in epigastric area that radiates to the shoulder, substernal area

Management of Pancreatitits

hydration, bed rest, analgesics, antidiabetic agents

Hepatitis

Hepatitis A: contaminated food, milk, water, feces

Hepatitis B: parenteral, sexual, oral, body fluid

Hepatitis C: blood or serum

Hepatitis D: similar to type B; only active in presence of HBV

Hepatitis E: Fecal oral route

Inflammation of liver tissue

fatigue, weight loss, right upper quadrant pain, pruritus

Management of Hepatitis

rest

small frequent meals

no alcohol

hydration

Appendicitis

inflammation of the appendix

mucosal ulceration, fecal mass

abdominal rigidity, anorexia, right lower quandrant pain

anorexia, nausea and vomiting, fever

Management of Appendicitis

NPO

hydration

bed rest

antibiotics

no heat to right lower quadrant(may rupture appendix)

Cholelithiasis

Stones in the gallbladder

Results from changes in bile composition

Stones are made of cholesterol and calcium or a mixture of both

Attacks follow meals rich in fats or at night

Right upper quandrant pain radiating to back and between shoulders

Nausea and vomiting

Management of Cholelithiasis

Fluid therapy, analgesic, antibiotics, and solbulizing agents (Actigal)

NCLEX Nuggets

Patients with GERD should sleep with the head of the bed elevated to reduce abdominal pressure

Sudden cessation of abdominal pain indicates perforation of an appendix

Patient should not eat for 6 to 12 hours before an endoscopy to ensure a clear view of GI tract

Fiber and residue are recommended in diet of diverticulitis

Abdominal rigidity is a classic sign of peritonitis

Hepatitis A is transmitted by ingestion of

   ontane contaminated food

Hepatitis B and C are transmitted by exposure to contaminated blood and blood products

A T-tube drains by gravity; not suction

Knowing when a person last ate before surgery is imperative to determine the type of anesthesia so that the chance of aspiration is minimized

Frequent stools are characteristic of Chron's Disease

Neomycin is given to decrease the bacterial content in the colon to prevent peritonitis before surgery

When cramping occurs while giving an enema, temporarily stop the flow of the solution

After a hemorrhoidectomy it is best to apply ice packs to the operative area, for the first 24 hours; heat causes vasodilation and could cause hemorrhaging.

After a liver biopsy it is best to position the patient on the right side; this will put pressure on it and reduce the chance of bleeding

Empty the bladder prior to a paracentesis so that the bladder will not get punctured.

Heartburn is the most common sign of hiatal hernia

GENITOURINARY SYSTEM NOTES

Acute Renal Failure

pre-renal, renal, post-renal

oliguric phase—urine output less than 400cc/day

diuretic phase—urine output is greater than 3 l/day

recovery phase urine output between 4 and 5l/day

Blood pressure affects regulation of the kidney's fluid volume

The Glomerular filtration rate is the rate at which the glomeruli filter blood. The normal rate is 120ml/min

The most accurate measurement of the GFR is the creatinine clearance

Dialysis—the passage of particles from an area of high concentration to low concentration

Peritoneal dialysis

hemodialysis

Benign Prostatic Hypertrophy

common in men over 50

enlargement of prostate gland

partial or complete obstruction of the urethra

urgency, frequency with alternating hesitancy during urination

nocturia

hematuria

retention

Pyelolithotomy—removal of stones from renal pelvis through flank incision

Percutaneous lithotripsy—endoscope is passed through a small incision made over the kidney to remove the calculi

Nephrectomy—removal of a kidney

Ureterolithotomy—incision in ureter to extract a stone

Nephrolithotomy—Parenchyma of a kidney is cut through a flank incision to remove a stone

T.U.R.P.—transurethral resection of the prostate

During peritoneal dialysis foul smelling outflow indicates peritonitis

A t-tube is used after a common bile duct until healing can occur

Pink-tinged blood is normal following a cystoscopy; bright red blood is not

A person in acute renal failure will be on a low sodium, low potassium, high carb diet

Continuous bladder irrigation removes clots from the bladder

Monitoring daily weights is the best way to assess hydration status.

Kidney Transplants

Implantation of a donated kidney after requiring dialysis during the last stage of renal disease

Immunosuppressive drugs 2 days before the transplant

Protective Isolation

Hemodialysis 24 hours before the transplant

Post-0p kidney transplant

Monitor cardiac and respiratory status, assess for organ rejection

Rejection usually occurs within 6 weeks; fever, malaise, anemia,

graft tenderness, oliguria

Avoid persons with infections for at least 3 months after surgery

TURP

Transurethral resection of prostate; excision of prostatic tissue in the urethra

CBI implemented

Hemodialysis

removes toxic wastes and other impurities from the blood

Peritoneal dialysis

removes toxins from the blood; uses the patient's peritoneal membrane as a semipermeable dialyzer.

Pyelonephritis

inflammation of the renal pelvis

bacterial infection causing cell destruction

fever, chills, N/V and flank pain

Fluids and antibiotics

Acute Renal Failure

inability of the kidneys to regulate fluid and electrolyte balance and remove toxic products

urine output less than 400ml/day for 1 to 2 weeks; weight gain, stupor; restrict fluid intake to amount needed to replace fluid loss

Chronic Renal Failure

progressive irreversible destruction of kidneys

3 Stages

first Stage: renal reserve is diminished, metabolic wastes do not accumulate

second stage: renal insufficiency occurs and metabolic waste accumulate

third stage; uremia occurs with decreased urine output

Benign Prostatic Hyperplasia

hyperplasia of the lateral and subcervical lobes of the prostate gland; enlargement of the structure

urgency, frequency and burning on urination, hesitancy and decreased force of stream

Manage with fluids, antibiotics and indwelling urinary catheter

NCLEX Nuggets

   Hyperkalemia is a common complication of acute renal failure

PSA is used as screening for prostatic cancer

A patient with calcium stones should follow an acid-ash diet

After a kidney transplant monitor the serum creatinine level

The kidneys maintain homeostasis of the blood by forming urine

Nephron is the functional unit of the kidney

The bladder has a holding capacity of 300-500cc of urine

A urinalysis can test for diabetes, dehydration and UTI

A urine culture and sensitivity can be collected by a clean catch specimen; or serile catherized specimen

A creatinine clearance test is the best indicator of the kidney's filtration function

Dysuria is burning during urination

Tenesmus are bladder spasms

During a parecentesis remove fluid slowly to decrease ascites

Struvite stones are infectious stones form with UTI

Foods high in purine should be avoided with patients who have uric acid stones

epididymitis includes scrotal pain, edema, n/v, and fever.

Steal syndrome develops from vascular insufficiency after a fistula

Pyelonephritis is an infectious disease causing inflammation of the kidney tissue. S/S are fever, chills, malaise, flank pain and costovertebral tenderness

Glomerulonephritis is a nonbacterial inflammation of the glomeruli in both kidneys; follows staph infection. S/S are fever, chills, nausea, vomiting, hematuria, elevated BUN and creatinine

Renal calculi (kidney stones) formed in the urinary tract causing pain and damage to tissue; consists of calcium, uric acid, and oxalates

Tenckhoff catheter is used in peritoneal dialysis

Absent bruit indicates nonpatent fistula

ENDOCRINE NOTES

Somogyi effect include in nightmares, sleep pattern disturbances and headaches

Ketoacidosis includes presence of ketones in the urine, kussmal respiration fruity odor breath

Cushing's Syndrome

weight gain, hyperglycemia, edema, muscle wasting, trunkal obesity, bruising buffalo hump

Addison's Disease (low levels of ACTH)

hypotension, weakness, lethargy, fatigue, and bronzing of the skin

Addisonian crisis includes dehydration, fever, hypotension, and electrolyte imbalances

The Hypothalmus controls temperature, blood pressure and respirations

Pituitary gland is the "master gland"; affects all hormone activity

Thyroid produces T4, T3, and thyrocalcitonin

Thyroidectomy

Removal of part or all of the thyroid gland

After surgery always check the surgical dressing for bleeding, especially at the back of the neck

Keep in semi-fowler's position

monitor V/S

Maintain seizure precautions

Assess for tetany

Assess for thyroid storm

Have calcium gluconate and tracheostomy tray at bedside

Monitor for Chvostek's and Trousseus's sign

Graves Disease

hyperthyroidism

heat intolerance, diaphoresis, tachycardia, palpitations, exophthalmoses ; avoid stimulants with caffeine

Monitor for thyroid storm (tachycardia, delirium, agitation, coma, death, dehydration, diarrhea)

Hypothyroidism

absence or decreased secretion of thyroid hormone

fatigue, weight gain, edema, cold intolerance, thick tongue, constipation

medication management includes : levothyroxine, liothyronine

Diabetes

Disturbance in the production, action, or rate of insulin use

Type I—usually develops in childhood; insulin dependent

Type II—usually develops after age 30; non insulin dependent

Insulin deprivation equals a decrease in glucose uptake

Low insulin triggers release of fatty acids that are not metabolized; then released as ketones in the blood and urine

Depression of protein synthesis

Assessment findings are polyphagia, polyuria, and polydipsia

  Diabetes Diet based on weight metabolic activities and personal activity levels

  Rapid-acting insulin (Lispro

  Short-acting insulin (Regular)

  Intermediate-acting (NPH)

  long-acting (Lantus)

Hypoglycemia

Nervousness, tremor, sweating, and hunger, night sweats,

Somogi Effect is rebound phenomenon occurring in diabetes after the over treatment with insulin induces hypoglycemia; this then produces hyperglycemia and ketosis

Hyperglycemia

Polyuria, polydipsia, and polyphagia

Diabetic Ketoacidosis

insulin deficiency and an increase in glucagon concentration

signs and symptoms are: abdominal pain, acetone breath, hot flushed skin, Kussmauls' respirations, Nausea and Vomiting and oliguria

Diabetes Insipidus

  deficiency of ADH(vasopressin)

  polyuria(5L/day or more)

polydipsia(4-40 L/Day)

Specific gravity less than 1.004; osmolality 50 to 200 mOsm/kg

Treat with ADH stimulants (Desmopressin)

Rotate insulin sites to prevent lipodystrophy

NCLEX Nuggets

Pancreas regulates glucose by secreting insulin

Diabetes Type I onset in younger population, requires insulin injections

Diabetes Type II onset in adults, overweight; insulin may be required

The peak of regular insulin is about 4 hours and lasts 5-7 hours

The peak for NPH insulin is about 8 hours and lasts 18 to 28 hours

Diaphoresis and shakiness are early signs of hypoglycemia

P's of diabetes are polyuria, polyphasia, polydipsia

If a patient becomes hypoglycemic mid-morning, this is caused by regular insulin, if it appears in the afternoon it is caused by NPH

When giving regular insulin and NPH, inject clear into cloudy or remember "RN", Regular to NPH.

Complications of Diabetes are foot ulcers, neuropathies

Hyperthyroidism is a hypermetabolic state with symptoms including anxiety, high blood pressure and tachycardia

Hypocalcemia includes symptoms such as muscle spasms, numbness, and tingling;treat with calcium gluconate

Cushing's syndrome results from excessive use of a glucocorticoid such as prednisone.

Diabetes insipidus is most prominent for deficient fluid volume.

A PTH deficiency would affect calcium and phosphorous levels

The presence of glucose in the nasal drainage indicate CSF leak

A patient who has an adrenalectomy requires steroids for life

Hypothyroidism produces coarse hair and alopecia

Hyperthyroidism produces weight loss and heat intolerance

MUSCULOSKELETAL NOTES

Amputation

removal of all or part of a limb

closed and open

elevate the affected extremity for 24 hours only

prevent hip flexion

monitor for hemorrhage

Laminectomy

Surgical excision of vertebral posterior arch

Assess neurovascular status

Turn the patient by logrolling

Prevent flexion of the neck

Muscle relaxants

Gout

inflammatory joint disease caused by the deposit of uric acid crystals; genetics

NCLEX Nuggets

Pressure on the heel and Achilles tendon could lead to nerve injury and foot drop

The four-point gait provides for the HIGHEST level of safety while using crutches

To minimize the side effects of ferrous sulfate give after meals

The typical look of a fractured hip is shortened, abducted, and externally rotated

Buck's traction is used to decrease pain by reducing muscle spasms.

The complication possible with a fracture of a long bone is a fat embolus

Compartment syndrome includes Pain, Paralysis, and Paresthesia

Crutch and Cane Walking

Two point gait—used for bilateral amputee with prosthesis

Three-point gait—used for non-weight bearing person with a fracture of the leg or hip

Four-point gait is used for patients affected by polio and cerebral palsy

Swing-to-gait used by the paraplegic with leg braces

REMEMBER: THE GOOD GO TO HEAVEN (move good leg first when going up)

THE BAD GO TO HELL (move crutches and bad leg first when going down)

Using crutches going up stairs, up with good leg, down with bad leg

Using crutches going down stairs, both crutches and bad leg down first, then good leg

Using a cane, hold cane on good side move cane and bad leg at the same time then good leg

Using a walker advance it and move into it

Use Buck's traction for femur or hip fracture

Bryant's traction is used for infants

5 P's of fractures are pain, pallor, pulselessness, parasthesia, and paralysis

Fat Embolism occurs in long bone fractures

After hip surgery maintain hips in abduction

limit hip flexion to 90 degrees when sitting

Do not cross legs

anticoagulants

Keep abduction pillow between legs at all times

INTEGUMENTARY NOTES

Skin Breakdown

Stage I: erythmea over bony prominences, blanches with pressure

Stage II: erythmea over bony prominences, does not blanch with pressure

Stage III:

ontanels

with blisters

Stage IV:

ontanels

beyond the epidermis and involves underlying structures

Burns

First degree: superficial (sunburn)

Second degree: dermal involvement (touching the stove)

Third degree: Muscle, bone gasoline explosions)

First degree burns show edema and blanching

Second degree burn wounds show fluid filled vesicles

Third degree burns show eschar

Rule of Nines

Head: 9%

Front: 18 %

Back: 18%

Arms :   18% (each arm is 9%)

Legs: 36% (each leg is 18%)

Perineum: 1% = 100%

A deep partial thickness burn is best treated with cool moist towels

Do not use ointments on burns

Myxedema is caused by decreased function of sebaceous glands

"ABCD" rule for monitoring skin lesions

A = asymmetry

B = border

C = color

D = diameter

NCLEX Nuggets

Petechia are flat red spots caused by capillaries that have broken

Vesicle is a fluid filled, elevated mass that measures less than 0.5 cm

Bleeding is a priority after a skin biopsy

Suspect inhalation injuries with soot in sputum

Varicella (chickenpox) has vesicles as the hallmark lesion

Tinea capitis is ringworm

MENTAL HEALTH NOTES

NCLEX Nuggets

Lithium toxicity S/S are lethargy, ataxia, slurred speech, tinnitus, severe nausea and vomiting, seizures, arrhythmias and hypotension

The "on-off" phenomenon appears in those with Parkinson Disease as a result of decreased effectiveness of Levodopa

Patient's with narcissistic personality display grandiosity, sense of entitlement

The best teaching for a patient with Parkinson disease is that of independence

Side effects of PCP are hallucinations and persecutory delusions

Side effects of Haldol are pill-rolling motions, drooling, and tremors

Patients with paranoid personality will use the defense mechanism projection

Delusion is false, fixed in belief and can't be changed with reasoning; grandeur, persecution, and ideas of reference

Hallucination are imaginery experiences which are not shared by anyone else

Illusions are misinterpretations of external stimuli

Paranoid character usually feels mistreated, suspicious, and mistrustful

Schizoid character socially uncommitted, cold, aloof

Schizotypal character has odd behaviors, bizarre thoughts, ideas of reference

Lithium is used in the treatment of mania and bipolar disorder (maintenance level is 0.6 to 1.5 meg/l Toxic level is greater than 1.5 meq/l side effects are fine tremors, nausea, diarrhea, fatigue and weight gain

Bipolar disorder is characterized by mood swings

Best intervention for Bipolar patients is to reduce distraction and encourage rest periods

Thorazine is used for hyperactivity in the bipolar patient

Akathisia may result within 6 hours of taking Haldol

When a patient focus on delusional activity you should refocus to reality

Borderline Personality characterisitics are those of engagement and rejection

The primary gain for a patient with anorexia is reduced anxiety and food control

A secondary characteristic of anorexia is amenorrhea

PHARMACOLOGY NOTES

Five Rights

Right drug

Right dose

Right route

Right time

Right patient

Always check for proper identification according to protocol

The *liver* is the primary organ for metabolizing drugs

Rotation of IV site is *72 hours*

Albuterol—bronchodilator, relieves bronchospasm

Allopurinol—antigout

Antabuse—alcohol ingestion

Aspirin—antipyretic; anti-inflammatory

Atropine—bradycardia

Benadryl—antihistamine

Catopril—antihypertensive

Congentin—antiparkinson disease

Calcium channel blockers—angina

Cephalosporins (ancef, Mefoxin, Keflex) broad spectrum antibiotic

Cimetidine—H2 receptor antagonist suppresses gastric acid

Diazepam—antianxiety; sedative

Dopamine—cardiogenic shock

Docusate sodium—stool softener

Epinephrine—used in cardiac arrest

Fentanyl—short acting analgesic

Gentamicin—antibiotic

Haldol—antipsychotic

Heparin—anticoagulant

Hydralazine—decreases blood pressure

Insulin—antidiabetic

INH—treatment of TB

Lactulose—constipation (diarrhea is sign of overdosage)

Mannitol—used with increased ICP

Monamine oxidase inhibitors (marpln, Nardil, Parnate);antidepressant

Meperdine hydrochloride—narcotic

Morphine—narcotic for severe pain

Narcan—opiate reversal

NSAIDS—pain relief, inflammation releief

Oxytocin—improves uterine contractions

Penicillian—antibiotic

Phenytoin—antiseizure

PTU—antithyroid hormone

Ranitidine—suppresses gastric secretions

Spironolactone—potassium sparing diuretic

Vancomycin—antibiotic

Warfin—anticoagulant (antidote is Vit K)

Beclomethasone is used in the treatment of asthma

Tensilon is used in the diagnosis of Myasthenia gravis

Diuretics reduce circulating blood volume

Pepcid diminishes gastric secretions in the stomach

Timoptic is instilled into the conjuctival sac for effectiveness

Major side-effects of *beta Blockers* are *bradycardia and bronchospasm*

NCLEX Nugget: BB=BB

NCLEX Nugget: when answering questions about medications to cluster responses into route; (PO,IV,SL) and know which one will be effective faster or slower

Safety measures should always be considered for when giving a sedative

Positive Inotropics increase contractility and Negative chronotropics decrease heart rate

The liver is the primary organ for metabolizing drugs

Antibiotics cause birth-control pills to be less effective

Clomide is usually first choice for infertility problems

Yutopar inhibits uterine contractions; decreases chance of premature labor

To avoid systemic absorption of eye medications hold slight pressure on the lacrimal sac for 1-3 minutes

Epinephrine is used in Emergencies

NCLEX Nugget: Always know the side effects and contraindications of your drugs!

OB-GYN NOTES

Nagele's rule: add 7 days to the first day of the last menstrual period and subtract 3 months

Signs of Pregnancy

Presumptive: amenorrhea, N/V, fatigue

Probable: Goodell's sign (softening of the cervix)

Chadwick's sign (blunesss of the vagina) ballottement, quickening

Positive: FHR by doppler, fetal movement felt by examiner

Nulligravida—never been pregnant

Primigravida-one pregnancy

Multigravida-more than one pregnancy

Nullipara-no birth at more than 20 weeks gestation

Primipara-one birth that occurred after 20th weeks of gestation

Multipara-more than one birth after 20th week of gestation

GTPAL

G = gravida; number of pregnancies

T = Term births

P = para; dead children

A = abortions

L = living children

Effacement-thinning of cervix

Dilation-opening of cervix

Lightening-fetal presenting part settles in the pelvic inlet

Amniotomy—the artificial rupture of membranes(AROM); increased risk of prolapsed cord

Episiotomy—incision of the perineal area

Lochia—vaginal discharge from the uterus

Lochia rubra—red in color; lasts 2-3 days

Lochia serosa—pinkish in color; lasts 3-10 days

Lochia alba—whitish in color; lasts 10-21 days

Umbilical Cord Care

Cord will fall off in 7-10 days

Cleanse daily with alcohol wipes

Sponge bath the newborn

Monitor for redness or yellow discharge around cord

Circumcision care

Plastibell

Do not use A & D ointment on the penis

Do not rub penis with wash cloth

Hogan

Apply A & D ointment 6 times daily

Monitor penis for bleeding

Abortions

Spontaneous-occurs naturally

Complete-all tissues and fetus are expelled

Incomplete-some parts of conception are expelled

Threatened-bleeding and/or cramping; no cervical dilation

Missed-the fetus dies

NCLEX Nuggets

Amniocentes is done at 15-18 week to detect genetic defects; AFP detects neural tube defects

Lightening is the dropping of presenting part into pelvis

Braxton Hicks are false labor contractions

Mother must void within 8 hours after delivery

Kegel exercises help strengthen the muscles around the perineal area

Pelvic tilt exercises help backache by strengthening the abdominal muscles

There are two arteries and one vein in the umbilical cord

Karotype is the picture after an amniocentesis

Primary sites for postpartum infection are endometrium, urinary tract and breasts

Uterine contractions occur at a rate of 1 contraction every 10 minutes or less

Signs and Symptoms of severe pre-eclampsia are blood pressure of 160/100 or higher and proteinuria of +2 or +3, severe headache, blurred vision, and photophobia

Seizure precautions are used for severe pre-eclampsia

Nulliparity is a risk for endometrial cancer

Pitocin is not given IV; it is given in a drip

If strong contractions occur over 90 seconds for a patient receiving Pitocin, stop the infusion and turn the patient on her side

Cervical ripening is the softening and thinning of the cervix

Labor has begun with regular progressive uterine contractions that increase with intensity

Betadine is an effective bactericidal compound

HELLP SYNDROME is characteristic of hemolysis, liver dysfunction, and low platelets

Vertex is when the presenting part has the flexed head entering the pelvis first

Lochia on postpartum day two should be deep red and thick

Breast feeding mothers should:

> Hold breast with four fingers along the bottom and thumb at the top, stimulate the rooting reflex then insert nipple and areola into the newborn's mouth, and put her finger into the newborn's mouth before removing breast

Assessement of a ruptured ectopic

> ontanels is a tender abdominal mass

Magnesium is given to treat pre-eclampsia

Hypotonic contractions usually occur during the ACTIVE phase of labor

When giving information to patients concerning abortion, the nurses answers should be based on facts and are unbiased in nature

Bonding between mother and baby is most effective right after birth

Heparin is used during pregnancy for anticoagulation therapy because its molecular size is too large to pass the placental barrier

Terbutaline sulfate reduces contractility; which then inhibits dilation and contractions. Terbutaline acts to arrest preterm labor

Laminaria tent is a safe and effective way of dilating the cervic

Ovulation occurs 14 days before the onset of menses

The rubin test determines the patency of fallopian tubes

A hysterosalpingogram helps to visualize the uterus and fallopian tubes and the pelvic organs for reproduction

Spontaneous abortions take place between 8-12 weeks of gestation

Placental formation is complete around the 12 week of pregnancy

Blood in the umbilical artery is more deoxygenated

Chadwicks's sign results from a purplish discoloration of the vaginal mucosa

Ladins sign is cervical softening

Hegar's sign is softening of lower uterine segment

Goodell's sign is softening of the cervix

The lecithin-sphingomyelin ratio helps determine the risk for RDS

An indirect coombs test test will test the mother's antibodies against RH-positive blood

A full bladder is required for the pregnant woman undergoing a ultrasound

Ambulation relieves Braxton-Hicks contractions; they increase when the patient is resting

Progressive dilation of the cervix is the most accurate indication of true labor

Fetal tones are best heard through the fetal back; position of ROP

(right occiput presenting)

Dilation and suction is used for early pregnancy termination

Rupture of membranes is a complication of amniocentesis

Leopold's maneuver is used to determine the position of the fetus

RPR (rapid plasma regain) screens for syphilis in the pregnant patient

Ritodrine is used to stop pre-term labor

Always massage the uterus for postpartum hemorrhage

Always shield the infant's eyes while undergoing lighting treatment for hyperbilirubinemia

Auscultate the fetal heart tones before and after an amniotomy so that changes can be noted

Erythromycin and silver nitrate used for prophylactic treatment of Neisseria Gonorrhoeae in newborns's eyes

PEDIATRIC NOTES

Erikson's Eight Stages

Trust vs mistrust	birth to 1 1/5 y.o.
Autonomy vs shame and doubt	1 1/5 to 3 y.o.
Initiative vs guilt	3 to 6 y.o.
Industry vs inferiority	6 to 12 y.o.
Ego identitiy vs role confusion	adolescence
Intimacy vs isolation	early adulthood
Generativity vs stagnation	middle age
Ego identity vs despair	later years

Croup

Barking cough, rib retractions, stridor, tachypnea

Croup tent

Humidified oxygen

Steroids for inflammation

Bronchiolitis

Usually preceded by upper respiratory infection, wheezing, congestion, nasal discharge, exposure to RSV

Patient on respiratory precautions

Otitis Media

Fever, pulling at ear

Antibiotics (give full course)

Cystic Fibrosis

Genetic

Positive sweat test

Affects pancreas, liver, and lungs

Pancreatic enzyme given with meals

Low-fat diet

Antibiotics

Bulging

fontanels are an indication of hydrocephalus

Increased ICP is shown in infants by irritability

When a child has meningitis, the inflammation can be spread to the cranial nerves resulting in loss of hearing

Vaso-occlusive crisis are the most frequent problem in children with sickle cell disease.

SIDS

In infant under 1 year of age

Cause unknown

Position on side or back for sleep

Epiglottitis

Child develops symptoms suddenly

Drooling, no swallowing, croaking inspiration

DO not assess pharynx; this can cause laryngospasm

NCLEX Nuggets

Amniotomy is used to enhance labor

Meconium is produced in first 24 hours from newborn

Sponge-bathe a newborn until umbilical cord stump falls off

Flaring nares in a newborn indicates respiratory distress

During phototherapy with an newborn the eyes should be covered with patches

Myelomeningocele is a neural tube defect that causes paralysis of the lower extremities

PKU after first feeding

PKU is an autosomal recessive gene

Vitamin K used for clotting in newborn

Obstruction of pancreatic duct and the absence of enzymes (trypsin, amylase, and Lipase) lead to failure to thrive

Compromised heart functioning in the infant often results in cyanosis and fatigue while sucking and swallowing because there is decreased cardiac output

Newborns with acquired herpes simplex virus type 2 infection often have visual acuity

Tetralogy of Fallot presents with clubbing of fingers

The Guthrie blood test detects abnormal PKU levels as early as 4 days of age

New foods should be initiated one at a time and continued for 4 to 5 days to assess for an allergic reaction

The American Academy of Pediatrics recommends the IM polio vaccine over the oral vaccine because it is safer

A side effect of vincristine is alopecia

Children with Leukemia most often die from infection

A side effect of Ritaline is anorexia; it should be given during meals

Choanal atresia is a lack of an opening between one or both of the nasal passages

The first indication of cystic fibrosis is meconium ileus

Snoring is expected in a child who just had a tonsillectomy

Mumps can cause orchitis in males(inflammation of the testes) and oophritis in females(inflammation of the ovaries)

Bradycardia is a sign of increased ICP

Elevation of the head helps increasing ICP

FLUID AND ELECTROLYTES NOTES

Water

Largest component in the body

Functions of Body Fluids

Transportation

Maintenance

Regulation

Third-spacing

Loss of extracellular fluid into a space that does not contribute to the balance of intracellular fluid and extracellular fluid Ex: ascities, burns, peritonitis, bowel obstruction

Lab Test for fluid monitoring

Osmolaity

osmolarity

Hypertonic solution

One solution is more concentrated than another; pulls fluid from another; contains more salt than normal cell (5% Dextrose Normal Saline) usage with cardiac or renal disease if they are unable tolerate the extra fluid watch for pulmonary edema.

Hypotonic solutions

One solution is more dilute than the other; forces fluid into another contains lower salt than normal cell (half-normal saline)

Isotonic solution

Equal amount of salt as normal cell (Lactated Ringer's)

Total Parenteral Nutrition

Used when the GI Tract for nutritional replenishment is inadequate

IV route

Infused by central line; superior vena cava or subclavian

Most Complication is sepsis; rebound hypoglycemia

Serum Values of Electrolytes

Cations	Concentration, mEq/L
Sodium	135-145
Potassium	3.5-4.5
Calcium	4.0-5.5
Magnesium	1.5-2.5

Anions

Chloride	95-105
CO_2	24-30
Phosphate	2.5-4.5

Hypokalemia

Deficits

Serum K = 3-4 is a 100-200 mEq deficit

2-3 is a 200-400 mEq deficit

Treatment

replacement 10 mEq/hr via peripheral IV

10 mEq α 0.1 mEq/L increase in serum K

Remember to check the Magmesium level

	Volume Deficit	
Symptoms	Moderate	Severe
Central Nervous System	Sleepiness Apathy Slow responsiveness Anorexia	Coma
Gastrointestinal System	Decrease in food intake	Nausea/Vomiting
Cardiovascular System	Tachycardia Orthostatic Hypotension	Absent pulses Hypotension Distant heart sounds
Tissue Signs	Decreased Turgor	Sunken eyes
Metabolism	Decreased Temperature	Significant temperature decrease
Renal	Oliguria	Anuria

	Volume Excess	
Symptoms	Moderate	Severe
Nervous System	Rare	
Gastrointestinal System	Edema	
Cardiovascular System	Increased CO Increased pulse pressure Distention of veins	Pulmonary Edema
Tissue Symptoms	Pitting Edema	Rales Vomiting
Metabolism	None	None
Renal	None	None

NCLEX Nuggets

Foods high in oxalate inhibit calcium absorption; beets, almonds, cocoa

Calcium gluconate can cause hypotension and cardiac dysrrhythmias

Potassium should not be given IV push or at infusion rates faster than 20meq per hour

KCL should be taken at meal time to decrease GI irritation

Edema is caused by sodium and water retention

DIAGNOSTIC TESTS

Computed tomography (CT) is a diagnostic procedure that uses special X-ray equipment to create cross-sectional pictures of your body. CT images are produced using X-ray technology and powerful computers.

The uses of CT include looking for

Broken bones

Cancers

Blood clots

Signs of heart disease

Internal bleeding

During a CT scan, you lie still on a table. The table slowly passes through the center of a large X-ray machine. The test is painless. During some tests you receive a contrast dye, which makes parts of your body show up better in the image.

Magnetic resonance imaging (MRI) uses a large magnet and radio waves to look at organs and structures inside your body. Health care professionals use MRI scans to diagnose a variety of conditions, from torn ligaments to tumors. MRIs are very useful for examining the brain and spinal cord.

During the scan, you lie on a table that slides inside a tunnel-shaped machine. Doing the scan can take a long time, and you must stay still. The scan is painless. The MRI machine makes a lot of noise. The technician may offer you earplugs.

Ultrasound uses high-frequency sound waves to look at organs and structures inside the body. Health care professionals use them to view the heart, blood vessels, kidneys, liver and other organs. During pregnancy, doctors use ultrasound tests to examine the fetus. Unlike x-rays, ultrasound does not involve exposure to radiation.

A liver biopsy is a procedure to obtain a sample of your liver tissue so that it can be examined under a microscope

After the biopsy, you will need to lie on your right side for a full two hours. This is done so that your weight puts pressure on the liver, reducing the chances of bleeding

A barium swallow, or upper GI series, is an x-ray test used to examine the upper digestive tract (the esophagus, stomach, and small intestine) You should drink more water than usual to help clear out the barium and to prevent constipation, which might be a side effect of the test. Your stool may appear light in color for a couple of days.

In colonoscopy, an endoscope is passed through the anus and all the way up through the entire colon (also called the large intestine) so that the doctor can see any abnormalities. Because you have been given a sedative, arrange for a friend or family member to drive you home afterward

Cystoscopy enables your doctor to take a direct look inside your bladder through a small camera inserted through the urethra

Angiography—an x-ray examination using contrast dye to visualize patency of arteries

Anigioplasty—Percutaneous transluminal coronary angioplasty (PTCA) is the introduction of a ballon-tipped catheter into the coronary artery to the stenosis to reduce or eliminate an occlusion

Bone Marrow Aspiration—collection of tissue from the bone marrow of the sternum

Bronchoscopy—a scope is placed down the mouth or nose to visualize the tracheobronchial tree;used to remove foreign body or obtain tissue specimen

Incentive Spirometry—assistive device used to open lungs to decrease pneumonia

Thoracentesis—removal of fluid or air from pleural space

REFERENCES

Anderson, D. L. (1997). *First Aid for the NCLEX-RN.* Stamford, Connecticut: Appleton & Lange.

Arnoldussen, B. (2008). *NCLEX-RN Medications You Need To Know For the Exam.* New York: KAPLAN PUBLISHING.

Hogan, M. A., & Madayag, T. (2004). *Medical-Surgical Nursing ; Reviews and Rationales.* Upper Saddle River, New Jersey: Pearson Prentice Hall.

Karch, A. M. (2009). *Lippincott's Nursing Drug Guide.* Philadelphia PA.: Lippincott Williams & Wilkins.

Linda Honan Pellico. (2008). *Medical-Surgical Nursing Made Incredibly Easy.* Philadelphia PA.: Lippincott Williams & Wilkins.

Michele Davidson, Marcia London, & & Patricia Ladewig. (2008). *Maternal-Newborn Nursing & Women's Health Across the Lifespan.* Upper Saddle River, New Jersey: Pearson Prentice Hall.

Mosby. (2006). *Mosby's Pocket Dictionary of Medicine, Nursing & Health Professions.* St. Louis, Missouri: Elsevier Publishing Inc.

Myers, E. (2003). *RNotes; Nurse's Clinical Pocket Guide.* Philadelphia PA.: F.A. Davis Company.

Pagna, K. D., & Pagana, T. J. (2006). *Mosby's manual of Diagnostic and Laboratory Tests.* St. Louis, Missouri: Elsevier Publishing Inc.

Saxton, D. F., Nugent, P. M., & Pelikan, P. K. (2006). *Mosby's Comprehensive review of Nursing for the NCLEX.* St. Louis, Missouri: Elsevier Publishing Inc.

Silvestri, L. A. (2006). *Q & A Review for the NCLEX-RN Examination.* St. Louis, Missouri: Elsevier Publishing Inc.

Smith, S. F. (2009). *Sandra Smith's Review for NCLEX-RN.* Sudbury, Ma: Jones and Bartlett Publishers.

Stuart, G. W. (2005). *Handbook of Psychiatric nursing.* St. Louis, Missouri: Elsevier Publishing Inc.

NUGGET NOTES

Nugget Notes

Nugget Notes